LARA WELLS

Chair Yoga for Seniors

Empowering Vitality at Every Stage of Life

First published by Lara Wells 2023

First edition

This book was professionally typeset on Reedsy.
Find out more at reedsy.com

Contents

INTRODUCTION

Lizzy, a senior living in a retirement community, stumbled upon this life-changing book. This guide introduced her to the gentle practice of chair yoga, designed for individuals with limited mobility. The book highlighted various physical and mental benefits, including improved flexibility, strength, balance, and reduced stress. Lizzy learned to prepare her space and mind for practice, and the book provided essential chair yoga poses and sequences to follow. Through breathwork and meditation techniques, Lizzy found inner peace and a renewed sense of vitality. Chair yoga transformed her life, proving that age was no barrier to feeling alive and embracing self-discovery.

Welcome to the world of chair yoga - a gentle and transformative practice that opens the door to well-being for people of all ages and abilities. As an experienced fitness coach, I have witnessed firsthand the incredible impact chair yoga can have on individuals, particularly seniors seeking to revitalize their mind, body, and spirit.

Chair yoga presents a unique opportunity for seniors to embark on a journey of self-discovery and holistic wellness without the constraints of traditional exercise forms. With a focus on nurturing the body through gentle movements and the mind through mindful breathwork, chair yoga allows seniors to embrace fitness on their own terms.

Through this practice, we explore the perfect harmony between motion and stillness, understanding that strength lies not only in muscles but in inner resilience and emotional balance. The benefits are abundant – from improved flexibility and balance, to reduced stress and enhanced relaxation.

In this transformative practice, the chair becomes a reliable companion, offering support and stability as we explore a range of poses that cater to individual needs and abilities. We adapt, modify, and customize each pose to ensure every senior feels empowered, safe, and fully engaged in their journey to well-being.

Through this guide, I will take you on a journey of self-exploration, sharing insights into the essence of chair yoga and its incredible potential to revitalize your mind, rejuvenate your body, and reconnect you with a sense of inner peace.

Whether you are a seasoned yoga enthusiast or completely new to the world of fitness, chair yoga welcomes you with open arms. Together, we will embrace this gentle approach to well-being, as I share my knowledge, experience, and passion for empowering seniors to lead a fulfilling and active life.

So, let's embark on this transformative path of chair yoga, where every breath, every stretch, and every moment brings us closer to a more vibrant and balanced version of ourselves. Get ready to experience the revitalizing benefits of chair yoga and rediscover the joy of movement, all from the comfort of your chair.

CHAPTER 1

Understanding Chair Yoga: A Gentle Approach to Well-being

Chair yoga is a modified form of yoga that adapts traditional yoga postures to be performed while sitting on a chair or using a chair for support. This gentle and accessible practice makes yoga accessible to people of all ages and abilities, including those with physical limitations, injuries, or balance issues. We will explore the essence of chair yoga, its benefits, key principles, and some simple exercises to get you started on your chair yoga journey.

1. **The Essence of Chair Yoga:**

Chair yoga retains the core elements of traditional yoga, focusing on breathing, gentle movements, and mindfulness. It promotes physical and mental well-being, aiming to improve flexibility, strength, balance, and overall body awareness. The primary difference lies in the use of a chair, which provides stability and support, making it suitable for seniors, individuals with mobility challenges, and anyone seeking a more relaxed approach to yoga.

2. **Benefits of Chair Yoga:**

a. *Increased Flexibility*: Chair yoga encourages gentle stretching, helping to increase flexibility and mobility in various body parts, such as the spine, hips, and shoulders.

b. *Improved Strength*: Despite being gentle, chair yoga postures engage muscles, leading to enhanced strength in the upper and lower body.

c. *Better Posture*: Practicing chair yoga can contribute to better posture by aligning the spine and promoting awareness of body alignment.

d. *Enhanced Balance*: The chair serves as a secure prop for balance-oriented poses, allowing individuals to work on their stability without fear of falling.

e. *Stress Relief and Relaxation*: Like other forms of yoga, chair yoga incorporates mindfulness and deep breathing techniques that aid in stress reduction and relaxation.

f. *Mind–Body Connection*: Chair yoga fosters a connection between the mind and body, enhancing self–awareness and mindfulness.

3. **Key Principles of Chair Yoga**:
   a. *Safety*: Chair yoga instructors prioritize safety by providing modifications and using props to accommodate individual needs and limitations.

b. *Mindful Breathing*: Focusing on breath work is an essential aspect of chair yoga, allowing participants to stay present and centered throughout the practice.

c. *Gentle Movement*: Chair yoga emphasizes slow, gentle movements that respect the body's limitations and capabilities.

d. *Adaptability*: Chair yoga can be tailored to meet the specific needs and goals of each participant, making it a versatile practice for diverse populations.

4. **Simple Chair Yoga Exercises**:
   a. *Seated Cat-Cow Stretch*: Sit on the chair with feet flat on the floor, hands on your knees. Inhale, arch your back, and lift your chest (Cow). Exhale, round your spine, and tuck your chin (Cat).

b. *Seated Twist:* Sit tall, cross your right hand over your left knee, and gently twist to the left. Take a few deep breaths, then switch to the other side.

c. *Seated Forward Bend*: Sit with your feet flat on the floor, inhale, and lengthen your spine. Exhale, hinge at the hips, and reach your hands towards your feet or the floor.

Getting Started with Chair Yoga: Your Path to Mindful Wellness

Embarking on a chair yoga journey can be an enriching experience, offering numerous benefits for both your body and mind. Whether you're new to yoga or have physical limitations that make traditional yoga challenging, chair yoga provides a gentle and accessible approach to the practice. In this guide, we'll explore the essential steps to help you get started with chair yoga, from finding the right class to setting up your practice space and understanding basic poses.

1. **Find the Right Class**:

If you're new to chair yoga, attending a class with an experienced instructor is highly recommended. Look for local community centers, yoga studios, or senior centers that offer chair yoga sessions. Choosing the right class ensures that you receive proper guidance, individual attention, and an opportunity to connect with like-minded individuals on the same journey.

2. **Gather the Necessary Equipment**:

One of the beauties of chair yoga is its minimalistic approach to equipment. You'll primarily need a sturdy and stable chair without wheels, armrests that don't slope downwards, and a backrest. Ensure the chair is the right height for you and provides ample support.

3. **Set Up Your Practice Space**:

Select a quiet and clutter-free space in your home where you can comfortably place your chair. Make sure you have enough room to move your arms and legs freely during the practice. Creating a calming atmosphere with soft lighting and perhaps some soothing music can further enhance your experience.

4. **Dress Comfortably**:

Put on something that is not too tight and is comfortable to move around in. Avoid clothes with restrictive waistbands or anything that might get in the way of your practice.

5. **Warm-Up and Mindful Breathing**:

Before diving into chair yoga poses, take a few minutes to warm up your body and focus on your breath. Sit comfortably on the chair, close your eyes, and take deep, slow breaths. Pay attention to each inhale and exhale, letting go of any tension or distractions.

6. **Basic Chair Yoga Poses:**

a. *Seated Mountain Pose*: Sit with a straight spine and feet firmly planted on the ground. Bring your hands to your lap, palms facing down. Take a deep breath and straighten your back, lifting your chest a bit. This pose helps establish a strong foundation for other movements.

b. *Seated Forward Fold*: Inhale, lift your arms overhead, and exhale as you fold forward from your hips, reaching towards your feet or the floor. This gentle stretch helps release tension in the spine and hamstrings.

c. *Seated Twist:* Sit tall, place your left hand on your right knee, and gently twist to the right.

Take a few deep breaths, then switch to the other side. Twisting helps improve digestion and spine flexibility.

d. *Seated Cat-Cow Stretch*: Rest your hands on your knees and inhale as you arch your back and lift your chest (Cow).

Take a deep breath and curl your back, bringing your chin in towards your chest (Cat). This movement promotes spinal flexibility.

7. **Practice Mindful Awareness:**

Throughout your chair yoga practice, maintain mindfulness and body awareness. Pay attention to how each movement feels in your body, and never force yourself into uncomfortable positions. Remember, chair yoga is about finding ease and comfort within the practice.

CHAPTER 2

Essential Chair Yoga Poses and Sequences for Holistic Well-being

Chair yoga offers a gentle and effective way to improve overall health and well-being without putting strain on the body. Whether you're a beginner or have experience with yoga, the following essential chair yoga poses and sequences will guide you on a journey of relaxation, strength, and mindfulness. These seated postures will target various muscle groups, enhance flexibility, and promote a deeper mind-body connection.

1. **Seated Mountain Pose:**
   - Sit comfortably with feet planted firmly on the ground.

- Align your spine, lift your chest, and relax your shoulders.

- Rest your hands on your knees with palms facing down.

- Close your eyes, breathe deeply, and find a sense of grounding and presence.

- Hold the pose for a minute, focusing on maintaining good posture and a steady breath.

Benefits: Seated Mountain Pose establishes a strong foundation, improves posture, and calms the mind.

2. **Seated Forward Fold:**
    - Inhale as you lift your arms overhead.

- Exhale and fold forward from your hips, reaching towards your feet or the floor.

- Allow your head and neck to relax, and let gravity gently stretch your back and hamstrings.

- Hold for several breaths, inhaling to lengthen your spine and exhaling to deepen the stretch.

Benefits: Seated Forward Fold releases tension in the spine, stretches the hamstrings, and promotes relaxation.

3. **Seated Twist:**
    - Position yourself upright with your feet firmly planted on the ground.

-Put your left hand on your right knee and slowly rotate your body to the right.

- Hold the backrest of the chair with your right hand for support.
    - Inhale to lengthen your spine, and exhale to deepen the twist.

- Take a few deep breaths, then switch sides and do the same.

Benefits: Seated Twists improve digestion, increase spine flexibility, and detoxify the body.

4. **Seated Chest Opener:**
    - Sit with a straight spine and feet flat on the floor.

- Clasp your hands behind your back, squeezing your shoulder blades together.

- Lift your chest and look up slightly, opening your heart.

- Take deep breaths, feeling the stretch in your chest and shoulders.

Benefits: Seated Chest Opener improves posture, expands the chest, and relieves tension in the shoulders.

5. **Seated Hip Opener:**
    - Sit with your feet hip-width apart and place your hands on your knees.

- Inhale and lift your right knee towards your chest.

- Hold your right ankle with both hands, gently pulling it towards your chest.

- Take a few deep breaths, then let go and switch to the other side.

Benefits: Seated Hip Opener increases hip flexibility and relieves tightness in the hips.

Chair Yoga Sequence for Stress Relief:

1. Seated Mountain Pose - 1 minute
2. Seated Forward Fold - 4 breaths
3. Seated Twist (each side) - 4 breaths per side
4. Seated Chest Opener - 4 breaths
5. Seated Hip Opener (each side) - 4 breaths per side
6. Mindful Breathing - 2 minutes

Gentle Warm-Up Poses: Preparing Your Body and Mind for Chair Yoga

A well-rounded chair yoga practice begins with gentle warm-up poses that help ease the body into movement and prepare the mind for the practice ahead. These warm-up poses serve to increase blood flow, lubricate joints, and release tension, ensuring a safe and enjoyable chair yoga experience. In this section, we will explore a selection of soothing warm-up poses that will help you transition into your chair yoga session with comfort and mindfulness.

1. **Seated Neck Stretch:**
   - Sit comfortably with a straight spine and feet flat on the floor.

- Inhale and lengthen your neck, reaching the crown of your head towards the ceiling.

- Exhale and gently tilt your head to the right, allowing your right ear to approach your right shoulder.

- Hold for a few breaths, feeling the stretch along the left side of your neck.

- Inhale to return to the center, and exhale as you tilt your head to the left.

- Repeat on each side for a total of 3-4 cycles.

Benefits: Seated Neck Stretch relieves tension in the neck and shoulders, promoting flexibility and relaxation.

2. **Seated Shoulder Rolls**:
   - Take a seat and rest your hands on your knees.

- Inhale as you lift your shoulders towards your ears.

- Exhale and roll your shoulders back and down, drawing shoulder blades together.
   - Repeat this movement for 5-6 rounds, then reverse direction, rolling your shoulders forward.

Benefits: Seated Shoulder Rolls help release shoulder tension and improve mobility in the shoulder joints.

3. **Seated Side Stretch:**
   - Maintain good posture by keeping your feet firmly planted on the ground.

- Inhale and reach your left arm overhead, extending through your fingertips.

- Exhale and lean to the right, stretching the left side of your body.

- Hold for a few breaths, feeling the lengthening sensation along the left side.

- Inhale to return to the center, and repeat on the other side.

- Perform 3-4 stretches on each side.

Benefits: Seated Side Stretch opens the sides of the body, enhances breathing, and relieves stiffness in the torso.

4. **Seated Ankle Circles**:
   - Find a comfortable position with your feet planted firmly on the ground.

- Lift your right foot off the ground and begin to make gentle circles with your right ankle.

- Perform 5-6 circles in one direction, then reverse the direction for another 5-6 circles.

- Lower your right foot to the floor, and repeat with the left foot.

Benefits: Seated Ankle Circles improve ankle flexibility, increase blood flow to the lower extremities, and promote balance.

5. **Seated Breath Awareness:**
   - Sit comfortably on the chair, close your eyes, and rest your hands on your knees.

- Take a few moments to take some deep breaths. Inhale through your nose and exhale through your mouth.

- Gradually shift your focus to your natural breath, observing its rhythm without attempting to change it.

- Stay in this state of mindful breath awareness for 2-3 minutes.

Benefits: Seated Breath Awareness helps center the mind, reduce stress, and cultivate mindfulness before the chair yoga practice.

Balancing and Strengthening Poses: Cultivating Stability and Vitality in Chair Yoga

Balancing and strengthening poses are integral components of a well-rounded chair yoga practice, offering numerous benefits for physical stability, muscle tone, and mental focus. These poses engage various muscle groups, enhance body awareness, and promote a sense of empowerment. In this section, we will explore a selection of balancing and strengthening poses specifically adapted for chair yoga, allowing individuals of all abilities to build strength, coordination, and confidence.

1. **Seated Warrior I:**
   - Sit tall with your feet hip-width apart and flat on the floor.

- Extend your right leg straight back, keeping your toes pointing forward.

- Bend your left knee, creating a 90-degree angle between your thigh and calf.

- Raise your arms overhead, palms facing each other or touching lightly.
   - Hold for 3-4 breaths, engaging your core and grounding through your seated position.
   - Repeat on the other side.

Benefits: Seated Warrior I strengthens the legs, stretches the hip flexors, and encourages a sense of inner strength and focus.

2. **Seated Warrior II:**
   - Sit tall with your feet hip-width apart and flat on the floor.

- Extend your right leg straight back and turn your right foot to the side.

- Bend your left leg, making sure it's in line with your ankle.

-Extend your arms out to the sides at shoulder level, with your palms facing downwards.

- Gaze over your left hand, maintaining a steady breath.

- Hold for 3-4 breaths, feeling the grounding sensation in your lower body.

- Repeat on the other side.

Benefits: Seated Warrior II enhances leg strength, opens the hips, and promotes balance and concentration.

3. **Seated Boat Pose:**
   - Position yourself at the front of the chair with your feet firmly on the ground.

- Use the sides of the chair for stability.

- Lean back a bit, engaging your abdominal muscles.

- Lift your feet off the floor, bringing your knees up to your chest.

- Find a balance point where you feel stable and hold for 5-6 breaths.

Benefits: Seated Boat Pose strengthens the abdominal muscles, improves posture, and cultivates a strong core.

4. **Seated Leg Lifts:**
   - Make sure you're sitting up straight with your feet firmly planted on the ground.

- Use the arms of the chair for stability.

- Inhale and lift your right leg off the ground, extending it straight out in front of you.

- Hold for a few breaths, engaging the quadriceps.

- Exhale as you lower the leg back down.

- Repeat on the other side for balanced strengthening.

Benefits: Seated Leg Lifts target the quadriceps, enhance lower body strength, and support stability.

5. **Seated Spinal Twist:**
   - Maintain good posture with your feet firmly planted on the ground.

- Inhale and lengthen your spine.

- Take a deep breath and slowly turn your body to the right, placing your left hand on your right knee and your right hand on the back of the chair.

- Hold for a few breaths, feeling the twist along the spine.

- Draw in a breath and come back to the middle, then do the same on the other side.

Benefits: Seated Spinal Twist improves spinal mobility, enhances digestion, and releases tension in the back and torso.

Relaxation Poses: Unwinding and Restoring in Chair Yoga

Relaxation poses are a crucial aspect of chair yoga that allows practitioners to unwind, let go of tension, and restore their mind and body. Incorporating these calming postures into your chair yoga practice provides a sanctuary of tranquility amidst the busyness of daily life. In this section, we will explore a collection of relaxing chair yoga poses that promote deep relaxation, reduce stress, and facilitate a state of inner peace.

1. **Seated Forward Bend with Support:**
   - Take a seat and make sure your feet are firmly planted on the ground.

- Place a pillow or cushion on your lap.

- Inhale and lengthen your spine.

- Exhale as you hinge forward from your hips, resting your upper body on the pillow.

- Allow your arms to hang loosely towards the floor or rest them on the pillow.

- Close your eyes and take slow, deep breaths as you surrender to the stretch.

Benefits: Seated Forward Bend with Support releases tension in the back and shoulders, calms the mind, and soothes the nervous system.

2. **Seated Child's Pose:**
   - Position yourself at the front of the chair with your feet firmly planted on the ground.

- Inhale and lengthen your spine.

- Exhale as you bend forward, bringing your torso between your thighs.

- Rest your forehead on your arms or on a cushion placed on your lap.

- Breathe deeply into your back, allowing it to expand with each breath.

Benefits: Seated Child's Pose gently stretches the lower back, hips, and shoulders, promoting relaxation and emotional release.

3. **Seated Heart Opener**:
   - Take a seat and make sure your feet are firmly planted on the ground.

- Interlace your fingers behind your back, opening your chest and drawing your shoulder blades together.

- Lift your arms slightly away from your back, opening the front of your chest.

- Breathe deeply into your heart space, feeling a sense of vulnerability and release.

Benefits: Seated Heart Opener fosters a feeling of emotional openness, relieves chest tightness, and encourages a sense of self-compassion.

4. **Seated Eagle Arms**:
   - Maintain good posture by keeping your feet firmly planted on the ground.

- Extend your arms straight in front of you at shoulder height.

- Cross your right arm over your left, bending your elbows, and bring the palms of your hands together.

- Raise your elbows while keeping your shoulders loose.

- Breathe deeply and hold the pose, feeling the gentle stretch across your upper back.

Benefits: Seated Eagle Arms alleviate tension in the shoulders and upper back, promoting a sense of lightness and ease.

5. **Seated Meditation**:
   - Take a seat and make sure your feet are firmly planted on the ground.

- Rest your hands on your knees, palms facing up or down.

- Close your eyes, or soften your gaze, and take slow, deep breaths.

- Bring your awareness to the present moment, letting go of any distractions.

- Focus on your breath, allowing it to anchor you in the here and now.

Benefits: Seated Meditation promotes mental clarity, relaxation, and a deeper connection to the present moment.

Chair Yoga Flows: Harmonizing Body, Breath, and Mind

Chair yoga flows are sequences of postures carefully crafted to create a fluid and seamless movement experience within the confines of a chair. These flows combine gentle stretches, strengthening poses, and relaxation techniques, allowing practitioners to reap the holistic benefits of yoga from a seated position. In this section, we will explore a variety of chair yoga flows that cater to different needs, from energizing morning sequences to calming evening flows.

1. **Energizing Morning Chair Yoga Flow:**
   This morning flow is designed to awaken the body, increase circulation, and set a positive tone for the day ahead.

a. *Seated Cat-Cow*:
   - Take a deep breath, arch your back, and raise your chest (Cow).

- Exhale, round your spine, and tuck your chin (Cat).

- Repeat this movement for 5-6 breaths, syncing breath with motion.

b. *Seated Twist*:
   - Inhale, lengthen your spine, and twist to the right, placing your left hand on your right knee and your right hand on the backrest.

- Exhale, deepen the twist, and hold for a few breaths.

- Take a deep breath and come back to the middle, then do the same on the other side.

c. *Seated Mountain to Forward Fold:*
    - Inhale, reach your arms overhead (Mountain).
    - Exhale, hinge forward from your hips, reaching towards your feet or the floor (Forward Fold).

- Inhale to return to the seated position, and repeat this flow 3-4 times.

d. *Seated Warrior I to Warrior II:*
    - Inhale, lift your right arm overhead, and stretch towards the left (Warrior I).

- Exhale, open your arms wide at shoulder height, and twist your torso to the left (Warrior II).

- Draw in a breath and come back to the middle, then do the same on the other side.

e. *Seated Sun Salutations:*
    - Inhale, lift your arms overhead (Mountain).

- Exhale, lower your hands to your heart center (Anjali Mudra).

- Repeat this sequence for 3-4 rounds, synchronizing breath with each movement.

2. **Balancing and Strengthening Chair Yoga Flow**:

This flow focuses on building strength, improving balance, and enhancing body awareness.

a. *Seated Warrior II to Warrior III:*
   - Inhale, bend your left knee and open your arms wide (Warrior II).

- Exhale, extend your right leg straight back, while leaning your upper body forward (Warrior III).

- Hold for a few breaths, engaging your core and balancing on your left foot.

- Inhale back to Warrior II, and repeat on the other side.

b. *Seated Eagle Arms to Leg Cross:*
   - Inhale, lift your right arm, and cross it over your left arm, entwining your forearms (Eagle Arms).

- Exhale, lift your right leg and cross it over your left leg, tucking your foot behind your calf (Leg Cross).

- Hold for 3-4 breaths, feeling the sense of balance and strength.

- Inhale back to the starting position, and repeat on the other side.

c. *Seated Boat Pose to Boat Twist:*
   - Inhale, lift your feet off the floor, finding a balance point (Boat Pose).

- Exhale, twist to the right, placing your left hand on the backrest and your right hand on your right knee (Boat Twist).

- Hold for a few breaths, engaging your core and maintaining stability.

- Inhale back to Boat Pose, and repeat on the other side.

3. **Calming Evening Chair Yoga Flow:**
   This gentle flow aims to relax the body, soothe the mind, and prepare for a peaceful night's rest.

a. *Seated Neck Stretch:*
   - Inhale, lengthen your neck, reaching the crown of your head towards the ceiling.

- Exhale, gently tilt your head to the right, allowing your right ear to approach your right shoulder.

- Hold for a few breaths, feeling the stretch along the left side of your neck.

- Draw in a breath and come back to the middle, then do the same on the other side.

b. *Seated Forward Bend with Support:*
   - Inhale, lengthen your spine.

- Exhale, hinge forward from your hips, resting your upper body on a cushion or pillow.

- Allow your arms to hang loosely towards the floor or rest them on the cushion.

- Close your eyes, and take slow, deep breaths as you surrender to the stretch.

c. *Seated Child's Pose:*
   - Inhale, lengthen your spine.

- Exhale, bend forward, bringing your torso between your thighs.

- Rest your forehead on your arms or on a cushion placed on your lap.

- Breathe deeply into your back, allowing it to expand with each breath.

d. *Seated Meditation*:
   - Take a seat in the chair and make sure your feet are firmly planted on the ground.

- Rest your hands on your knees, palms facing up or down.

- Close your eyes, or soften your gaze, and take slow, deep breaths.

- Bring your awareness to the present moment, letting go of any distractions.

- Focus on your breath, allowing it to anchor you in the here and now.

CHAPTER 3

Breathwork and Meditation Techniques: Cultivating Calmness and Inner Awareness in Chair Yoga

Breathwork and meditation are integral components of chair yoga, offering profound benefits for stress reduction, emotional well-being, and mental clarity. These techniques allow practitioners to connect with their inner selves, find tranquility, and deepen their mind-body connection. In this section, we will explore various breathwork and meditation techniques specifically adapted for chair yoga, empowering individuals to discover the transformative power of their breath and cultivate a peaceful mind.

1. **Diaphragmatic Breathing (Belly Breathing):**
    - Place your feet flat on the floor in a comfortable chair.

- Put one hand on your tummy, the other on your chest.

- Take a deep breath in through your nose, allowing your stomach to puff out like a balloon.

- Slowly exhale through your mouth, allowing your tummy to sag slightly.

- Focus on the sensation of your breath, directing it deep into your belly.

- Practice this technique for 2-3 minutes, calming the nervous system and promoting relaxation.

Benefits: Diaphragmatic Breathing promotes deep relaxation, reduces stress, and increases oxygen intake, leading to a sense of calmness and grounding.

2. **4-7-8 Breathing (Relaxing Breath):**
   - Sit comfortably with your feet flat on the ground and your back straight.

- Take a four-count calm inhalation via your nose.

- Hold your breath for a count of 7.

- Exhale completely and audibly through your mouth for a count of 8.

- Repeat this cycle for 4-5 rounds, gradually extending the breath counts if comfortable.

Benefits: 4-7-8 Breathing calms the mind, reduces anxiety, and helps in falling asleep or managing stressful situations.

3. **Alternate Nostril Breathing (Nadi Shodhana):**
   - Sit comfortably, and with your right thumb, close off your right nostril.

- Take a long, slow breath in through your left nostril.

- Close off your left nostril with your right ring finger and release your right nostril.

-Exhale via your right nostril fully and easily.

- Inhale deeply through your right nostril, then close it off again.

- Open your left nostril and breathe out through it.

- This completes one round. Continue for 5-7 rounds.

Benefits: Alternate Nostril Breathing balances the left and right sides of the brain, calms the nervous system, and enhances mental clarity.

4. **Loving-Kindness Meditation (Metta):**
   - Take a comfortable seat, close your eyes, and place your hands on your knees.

- Begin by sending feelings of love and kindness to yourself, silently repeating phrases like "May I be happy, may I be peaceful, may I be safe."

- Then, extend these well-wishes to others, starting with a loved one, and eventually including neutral and challenging individuals.

- Continue to silently repeat the phrases, embracing a sense of compassion and goodwill towards all beings.

Benefits: Loving-Kindness Meditation cultivates feelings of empathy, compassion, and interconnectedness, promoting emotional well-being and reducing negativity.

5. Mindfulness Meditation:
   - Sit comfortably with your back straight and your feet flat on the floor.

- Bring your attention to your breath, focusing on the sensation of each inhalation and exhalation.

- If thoughts or distractions arise, simply acknowledge them without judgment and gently guide your attention back to your breath.

- Practice mindfulness meditation for 5-10 minutes, gradually extending the duration as you feel more comfortable.

Benefits: Mindfulness Meditation enhances present-moment awareness, reduces stress, and fosters a deeper connection to oneself and the surrounding environment.

Mindful Breathing: Harnessing the Power of the Present Moment in Chair Yoga

Mindful breathing is a fundamental aspect of chair yoga that involves bringing focused awareness to the breath, fostering a profound connection between body and mind. This simple yet powerful practice allows practitioners to anchor themselves in the present moment, alleviating stress, promoting relaxation, and cultivating mindfulness. In this section, we will explore the essence of mindful breathing in chair yoga, its benefits, and various techniques to help you embark on a journey of self-awareness and inner peace.

1. The Essence of Mindful Breathing:
   Mindful breathing, also known as conscious or focused breathing,

centers on paying attention to the breath as it flows in and out of the body. It encourages non-judgmental awareness of the present moment, without attachment to the past or future. By bringing our attention to the breath, we create a sense of grounding and a doorway to deeper self-awareness.

2. **Benefits of Mindful Breathing in Chair Yoga:**
   a. *Stress Reduction*: Mindful breathing triggers the body's relaxation response, reducing the production of stress hormones and inducing a sense of calmness.

b. *Enhanced Focus*: By directing our attention to the breath, we train our minds to stay present, leading to improved concentration and mental clarity.

c. *Emotional Regulation*: Mindful breathing helps us observe and understand our emotions without immediate reactions, allowing for more measured responses to challenging situations.

d. *Improved Self-Awareness*: As we become more attuned to our breath, we gain insight into our thought patterns, physical sensations, and emotional states.

e. *Lower Blood Pressure*: Regular practice of mindful breathing has been linked to reduced blood pressure levels, benefiting cardiovascular health.

3. **Mindful Breathing Techniques:**

a. *Breath Awareness:*
   - Sit comfortably with your feet flat on the floor and your hands resting on your knees.

- Shield your gaze or avert your eyes.

- Bring your attention to your breath, noticing the sensation of the air entering and leaving your nostrils or the rise and fall of your abdomen.

- Don't try to regulate your breath; just let it happen naturally.

- Whenever your thoughts stray, gently nudge them back to your breathing.

b. *Counted Breathing*:
 -To the count of four, slowly inhale through your nostrils.

- Wait four counts before you breathe.

- Exhale slowly through your nose or mouth to a count of six.

- Pause briefly for a count of two before beginning the next breath cycle.

- Continue this pattern for several rounds, adjusting the counts to suit your comfort.

c. *Square Breathing*:
 - To the count of four, slowly inhale through your nostrils.

- Wait four counts before you breathe.

- Exhale completely to a count of four.

- Pause briefly for a count of four before starting the next breath cycle.

- Repeat this pattern for several rounds, creating a balanced and calming rhythm.

4. **Integrating Mindful Breathing into Chair Yoga:**

Mindful breathing can be practiced at any time during your chair yoga routine. Begin each session with a few minutes of breath awareness to center yourself and set an intention for your practice. You can also incorporate mindful breathing during asanas (poses), focusing on your breath to stay present and deepen your stretches. End each session with a few minutes of breath awareness or a guided meditation to fully absorb the benefits of your chair yoga practice.

Relaxation Techniques: Unwinding the Mind and Body in Chair Yoga

Relaxation techniques are a vital component of chair yoga, providing practitioners with invaluable tools to release tension, calm the mind, and promote a state of deep relaxation. These practices allow individuals of all abilities to experience the transformative benefits of relaxation without the need for strenuous physical postures. In this section, we will explore a range of relaxation techniques specifically tailored for chair yoga, offering you the opportunity to unwind, rejuvenate, and find inner serenity.

1. **Progressive Muscle Relaxation:**

Progressive Muscle Relaxation (PMR) is a systematic technique that involves tensing and then releasing different muscle groups in the body. This practice promotes physical relaxation and heightened body awareness.

- Sit comfortably on the chair with your eyes closed.

- Start with your feet, tensing the muscles in your toes and feet for a few seconds.

- Release the tension and let your feet and toes fully relax.

- Move up to your calves, thighs, abdomen, chest, arms, and shoulders, repeating the process for each muscle group.

- Finally, tense the muscles in your face, including your jaw, forehead, and cheeks, before releasing the tension.

- Take a few deep breaths, embracing the sense of relaxation throughout your body.

Benefits: Progressive Muscle Relaxation reduces muscle tension, eases physical discomfort, and induces a deep state of relaxation.

2. **Guided Imagery:**

Guided imagery is a relaxation technique that involves visualizing peaceful and calming scenarios to evoke positive emotions and reduce stress.

- Sit comfortably on the chair with your eyes closed.

- To regain your composure, take a few long breaths.

- Imagine a serene and beautiful place, such as a beach, forest, or meadow.

- Visualize yourself in this tranquil setting, paying attention to the sounds, smells, and colors around you.

- Engage your senses and immerse yourself in the calming experience.

- Spend a few minutes in this peaceful imagery, allowing it to envelop you with a sense of tranquility.

Benefits: Guided Imagery promotes relaxation, reduces anxiety, and fosters a positive state of mind.

3. **Autogenic Relaxation**:
   Autogenic Relaxation is a self-guided technique that involves repeating affirmations to induce a state of deep relaxation and calmness.

- Sit comfortably on the chair with your eyes closed.

- Inwardly repeat positive and relaxing phrases to yourself, such as "I am calm and peaceful" or "I am safe and at ease."

- As you repeat the phrases, focus on experiencing the feelings of calmness and relaxation within your body and mind.

- Continue to affirm these positive statements for several minutes, allowing them to soothe your entire being.

Benefits: Autogenic Relaxation cultivates a sense of inner peace, reduces stress, and enhances self-awareness.

4. **Breath Awareness Relaxation:**
   Breath Awareness Relaxation is a simple and effective technique that centers on observing the natural rhythm of your breath to create a state

of relaxation.

- Place your feet flat on the ground and take a comfortable seat in the chair.

- Shift your focus or avert your gaze.

- Bring your awareness to your breath, noticing the gentle inhales and exhales.

- Avoid controlling or altering your breath; simply observe it with a sense of non-judgmental presence.

- Allow your body to relax with each breath, feeling tension dissipate with every exhalation.

- Stay in this state of mindful breath awareness for several minutes, embracing the tranquility it brings.

Benefits: Breath Awareness Relaxation calms the mind, reduces stress, and promotes a sense of centeredness.

5. **Aromatherapy Relaxation:**

Aromatherapy Relaxation involves the use of essential oils or scents to create a soothing and calming atmosphere during chair yoga practice.

- Sit comfortably on the chair with your eyes closed.

- Use a diffuser or a few drops of essential oil on a cotton ball placed nearby to release a calming scent into the air.

- Inhale deeply, focusing on the aroma and its impact on your senses.

- Let the scent envelop you, allowing it to transport you to a place of relaxation and peace.

Benefits: Aromatherapy Relaxation enhances the relaxation experience, reduces stress, and supports emotional well-being.

Combining Breath and Movement: Flowing with Grace in Chair Yoga

Combining breath and movement is at the heart of chair yoga, creating a harmonious and meditative flow that fosters a deeper mind-body connection. This practice allows practitioners to embrace the fluidity of their breath while moving gracefully through gentle postures, enhancing flexibility, mindfulness, and overall well-being. In this section, we will explore the essence of combining breath and movement in chair yoga, its benefits, and techniques to help you embark on a journey of seamless and mindful practice.

1. **The Essence of Combining Breath and Movement:**
   In chair yoga, the synchronization of breath with movement brings intention and awareness to each posture. The breath serves as a guide, allowing practitioners to move with grace and mindfulness, creating a meditative and calming experience. By uniting breath and movement, we cultivate a sense of presence, flow, and self-attunement.

2. **Benefits of Combining Breath and Movement in Chair Yoga:**
   a. *Mindfulness*: By coordinating breath with movement, we anchor our attention in the present moment, fostering a deep state of mindfulness.

b. *Improved Body Awareness*: The integration of breath and movement enhances our sensitivity to the body's alignment, improving posture and reducing the risk of injury.

c. *Stress Reduction*: The rhythmic flow of breath and movement induces the body's relaxation response, reducing stress and tension.

d. *Enhanced Flexibility*: Coordinating breath with movement allows for deeper stretches and greater range of motion.

e. *Emotional Balance*: The union of breath and movement encourages emotional regulation and cultivates a sense of tranquility.

3. **Techniques for Combining Breath and Movement in Chair Yoga:**
   a. *Flowing Breath with Gentle Stretches*:
   - Inhale deeply through the nose as you reach your arms overhead.

- Exhale slowly through the mouth as you lower your arms and hinge forward from your hips, performing a gentle forward bend.

- Inhale, lengthen your spine, and return to the seated position.

- Repeat this flow for several rounds, connecting your breath with the movement.

b. *Breath-Coordinated Shoulder Circles*:
   - Relax in a chair with your feet flat on the ground.

- Inhale as you lift your shoulders towards your ears.

- Exhale and roll your shoulders back and down, drawing shoulder blades together.

- Continue this movement in a circular motion, coordinating each circle with a full breath cycle.

c. *Flowing Warrior I to Warrior II:*
   - Take a deep breath in, extend your arms upwards, and join your fingers.

- Exhale, release your hands and stretch them out to the sides at shoulder height, opening into Warrior II.

- Inhale back to Warrior I, and repeat the flow for several rounds, coordinating each transition with your breath.

d. *Breath-Coordinated Spinal Twists:*
   - Put your feet flat on the ground and take a comfortable seat.

- Inhale as you lengthen your spine.

- Exhale and twist to the right, placing your left hand on your right knee and your right hand on the backrest.

- Inhale back to the center, and repeat the twist on the other side.

4. Embracing Mindful Flow in Chair Yoga:
   To embrace a mindful flow in chair yoga, remember the following principles:

a. *Connect*: Create a conscious connection between your breath and each movement, fostering awareness and intention.

b. *Breathe Naturally:* Allow your breath to flow naturally and without force, embracing the pace that feels comfortable for you.

c. *Move Gracefully:* Move with gentleness and fluidity, honoring the limitations of your body and allowing for modifications as needed.

d. *Be Present*: Stay present in the flow, observing your body's sensations and your breath's rhythm as you move through the postures.

CHAPTER 4

Chair Yoga for Specific Needs and Conditions: Adapting the Practice for Individual Well-being

Chair yoga is a versatile and inclusive practice that can be adapted to meet the specific needs and conditions of individuals with varying abilities and limitations. Whether managing chronic conditions, recovering from injuries, or seeking gentle exercise, chair yoga offers a safe and accessible way to experience the benefits of yoga from a seated position. In this section, we will explore how chair yoga can be tailored to cater to specific needs and conditions, empowering individuals to embrace the healing potential of this adaptable practice.

1. **Chair Yoga for Seniors:**

Chair yoga is especially beneficial for seniors, offering gentle movement and stretching that cater to aging bodies and reduced mobility. It provides an opportunity for seniors to stay active, improve flexibility, and maintain joint health without the strain of traditional yoga postures.

- *Gentle Warm-Up:* Start with gentle neck, shoulder, and wrist movements, gradually transitioning to seated twists and side stretches.

- *Joint Mobility:* Incorporate circular movements for ankles, knees, and hips to enhance joint mobility and reduce stiffness.

- *Balance Practice*: Include seated balance poses, such as seated tree pose or knee lifts, to improve stability and reduce the risk of falls.

- *Breathing Techniques*: Focus on breath awareness and relaxation techniques to promote mental clarity and emotional well-being.

2. **Chair Yoga for Office Workers:**
Chair yoga offers office workers a valuable opportunity to combat the adverse effects of prolonged sitting, such as back pain and muscle tension. Incorporating chair yoga into the workday can enhance productivity, reduce stress, and increase overall well-being.

- *Neck and Shoulder Relief:* Integrate neck rolls, shoulder shrugs, and seated shoulder stretches to release tension accumulated from desk work.

- *Seated Forward Folds:* Promote spinal flexibility and alleviate lower back discomfort by practicing gentle seated forward folds.

- *Wrist and Hand Exercises*: Include wrist circles and finger stretches to prevent repetitive strain injuries caused by typing and mouse usage.

- *Mindful Breaks:* Encourage taking short breaks throughout the day for mindful breathwork and relaxation, enhancing focus and productivity.

3. **Chair Yoga for Individuals with Limited Mobility:**
Chair yoga is a perfect option for individuals with limited mobility, such as those recovering from surgeries or living with physical disabili-

ties. It provides an opportunity to strengthen and stretch muscles while being seated or using the chair for support.

- *Gentle Joint Exercises*: Focus on range-of-motion exercises for the neck, shoulders, elbows, hips, knees, and ankles to maintain joint health and flexibility.

- *Seated Strength Poses:* Incorporate seated leg lifts, seated twists, and core-strengthening exercises to build muscle strength without standing.

- *Chair-Assisted Stretches*: Use the chair for support in performing stretches like seated hamstring stretches and chest openers.

- *Mindful Meditation:* Introduce seated mindfulness meditation for relaxation and stress reduction, creating a sense of ease and well-being.

4. **Chair Yoga for Stress Relief:**
   Chair yoga serves as a powerful tool for stress relief, as it combines breathwork, gentle movements, and relaxation techniques to promote calmness and inner balance.

- *Deep Breathing*: Practice various breathwork techniques, such as diaphragmatic breathing and 4-7-8 breathing, to activate the body's relaxation response.

- *Restorative Poses:* Integrate restorative postures, such as supported forward bends and heart openers, to induce relaxation and release tension.

- *Guided Relaxation*: Offer guided imagery or body scan meditation to help individuals unwind and find peace within.

- *Mindful Awareness*: Encourage present-moment awareness during the practice, focusing on the sensations of the breath and body to foster mindfulness.

Yoga for Arthritis: Gentle and Therapeutic Practices for Joint Health

Yoga has shown to be a valuable complementary therapy for individuals living with arthritis, a condition characterized by joint inflammation and pain. The gentle and therapeutic nature of yoga can help improve joint flexibility, reduce stiffness, and enhance overall well-being. In this section, we will explore how yoga can be adapted specifically for arthritis, offering a safe and effective way to manage symptoms, promote joint health, and improve the the condition's impact on the quality of life for individuals afflicted.

1. **Understanding Arthritis:**

Arthritis refers to a group of more than 100 conditions that affect the joints, causing pain, stiffness, and swelling. Rheumatoid arthritis and osteoarthritis are the two most prevalent kinds of arthritis. While arthritis can be a chronic and debilitating condition, adopting a holistic approach that includes yoga can be beneficial in managing its impact on daily life.

2. **Benefits of Yoga for Arthritis:**

a. *Joint Mobility:* Gentle yoga movements help lubricate the joints, reducing stiffness and promoting mobility.

b. *Muscle Strength*: Yoga poses that engage the muscles gently build strength, supporting the joints and improving stability.

c. *Mind-Body Connection:* Mindfulness practices in yoga promote relaxation and reduce stress, which can alleviate arthritis-related tension.

d. *Pain Management*: Yoga encourages the release of endorphins, the body's natural painkillers, helping to manage arthritis-related discomfort.

e. *Improved Sleep:* Regular yoga practice can lead to better sleep quality, which is essential for overall health and well-being.

3. **Adapted Yoga Practices for Arthritis**:
   a. *Gentle Warm-Up:*
   - Start with gentle joint warm-ups, such as wrist circles, ankle rotations, and neck stretches, to prepare the body for movement.

b. *Seated Poses*:
   - Focus on seated poses, such as Seated Mountain Pose, Seated Forward Bend, and Seated Twist, to avoid stress on weight-bearing joints.

c. *Restorative Poses:*
   - Incorporate restorative poses, like Supported Child's Pose and Reclining Bound Angle Pose, using props for added comfort and support.

d. *Joint-Friendly Movements:*
   - Emphasize gentle and slow movements to prevent excessive strain on the joints, promoting a safe and sustainable practice.

e. *Modified Sun Salutations:*
   - Adapt Sun Salutations to avoid putting pressure on the wrists and

knees, replacing Chaturanga Dandasana with Knee-to-Chest Pose and Cobra with Sphinx Pose.

4. **Breathing Techniques and Meditation**:
   a. *Breathwork*:
   - Practice diaphragmatic breathing or 4-7-8 breathing to induce relaxation and reduce stress, which can exacerbate arthritis symptoms.

b. *Meditation*:
   - Engage in mindfulness meditation to cultivate a positive outlook and manage the emotional aspects of living with arthritis.

5. **Listen to Your Body:**
   It's critical to pay attention to your body's signals and stay in your comfort zone. If a pose causes pain or discomfort, modify it or skip it altogether. Yoga is not about pushing your limits but rather finding a gentle balance that promotes healing and well-being.

6. **Seek Guidance:**
   If you're new to yoga or living with arthritis, consider seeking guidance from a qualified and experienced yoga instructor who can tailor the practice to your specific needs and limitations. They can provide personalized modifications and ensure that the practice is safe and suitable for you.

Osteoporosis and Bone Health: Gentle Strength and Flexibility for Stronger Bones

Chair yoga offers a gentle and accessible way for individuals with osteoporosis to improve bone health, build strength, and enhance flexibility. Osteoporosis, a condition characterized by low bone density and increased risk of fractures, requires exercise that is safe and supportive for the bones. Chair yoga provides a modified practice that can be done while seated or using a chair for support, making it suitable for those with limited mobility or balance issues. In this section, we will explore how chair yoga can benefit individuals with osteoporosis and provide a series of safe and effective chair yoga poses to promote bone health and overall well-being.

1. **The Importance of Bone Health:**
   For general health and quality of life, maintaining bone health is essential. Osteoporosis can lead to weakened bones, increasing the risk of fractures and impacting daily activities and mobility.

2. **Understanding Chair Yoga for Osteoporosis**:
   Chair yoga adapts traditional yoga poses for a seated or supported practice, making it safe and effective for individuals with osteoporosis. The practice focuses on gentle stretches, strengthening movements, and breathwork to enhance bone health, balance, and flexibility.

3. **Chair Yoga Poses for Osteoporosis and Bone Health:**
   a. *Seated Mountain Pose*:
   - Sit upright on a chair, your feet flat on the ground.

-Your head, neck, and spine should be in a straight line.

- Relax your shoulders and place your hands on your thighs or in a comfortable position on your lap.

- Breathe deeply and hold the pose for a few breaths, focusing on elongating your spine and engaging your core muscles.

b. *Seated Twist:*
   - Put your feet flat on the ground and take a seat comfortably.

- Inhale and lengthen your spine.

- Exhale and twist to the right, placing your left hand on the outside of your right knee and your right hand on the backrest of the chair.

- Inhale back to center, and then exhale, twisting to the left.
   - Continue alternating sides for several rounds, gently massaging the spine and promoting better flexibility.

c. *Seated Forward Bend:*
   - Place your feet flat on the floor and occupy the chair.

- Inhale and lengthen your spine.

- Exhale and hinge forward from your hips, reaching your hands towards your feet or the floor.

- Inhale as you lengthen your spine again, and then exhale, folding forward a bit deeper.

- Hold the pose for a few breaths, feeling the gentle stretch along the spine and hamstrings.

d. *Seated Cat-Cow Stretch:*

 - Sit tall with your feet flat on the floor.

- Inhale and arch your back, lifting your chest and chin (Cow Pose).

- Exhale and round your back, tucking your chin towards your chest (Cat Pose).

- Continue flowing between Cow and Cat Poses, focusing on the movement of your spine and breathing deeply.

4. **Safety Considerations:**
   When practicing chair yoga for osteoporosis, it's essential to prioritize safety and avoid movements that may put excessive pressure on the spine or risk of falls. Avoid deep forward bends, twists, or poses that involve rounding the spine.

5. **Breathing and Mindfulness**:
   Incorporate mindful breathing techniques into your chair yoga practice to promote relaxation and reduce stress. Focus on your breath during each pose, inhaling deeply and exhaling fully to enhance the mind-body connection.

6. **Consistency and Progression**:
   Consistent chair yoga practice is key to experiencing the benefits for bone health. Gradually progress in your practice, exploring deeper stretches and building strength over time.

Managing Chronic Pain: Finding Relief and Empowerment in Gentle Movements

Chronic pain can significantly impact daily life, making it challenging to engage in regular physical activities. However, chair yoga offers a safe and accessible way for individuals dealing with chronic pain to find relief, improve flexibility, and cultivate a sense of empowerment. By adapting traditional yoga poses for a seated or supported practice, chair yoga provides gentle movements that can be modified to suit individual needs and limitations. In this section, we will explore how chair yoga can be a valuable tool for managing chronic pain and enhancing overall well-being.

1. **Understanding Chronic Pain:**
   Chronic pain is persistent pain that lasts for an extended period, often beyond three months. It can be caused by various conditions, such as arthritis, fibromyalgia, back pain, or injuries.

2. **The Benefits of Chair Yoga for Chronic Pain**:
   Chair yoga offers numerous benefits for individuals managing chronic pain:

- *Gentle Movements:* Chair yoga incorporates slow and gentle movements that are less likely to strain muscles or exacerbate pain.

- *Increased Flexibility:* Regular chair yoga practice can improve flexibility, reducing stiffness and discomfort in the body.

- *Mindfulness and Relaxation*: The practice of chair yoga emphasizes mindfulness and relaxation techniques, promoting a sense of calm and reducing stress-related pain.

- *Empowerment*: Chair yoga can empower individuals to feel more in control of their bodies and their pain, fostering a positive outlook.

3. **Chair Yoga Poses for Managing Chronic Pain**:
   a. *Seated Neck Rolls:*
   - Sit tall on the chair with your feet flat on the floor.

- Inhale and lengthen your spine.

- Exhale and gently drop your chin towards your chest, rolling your neck from side to side.

- Continue this movement for a few rounds, releasing tension in the neck and shoulders.

b. *Seated Spinal Twist:*
   - Take a comfortable seat with your feet flat on the ground.

- Inhale and lengthen your spine.

- Exhale and twist to the right, placing your left hand on the outside of your right knee and your right hand on the backrest of the chair.

- Inhale back to center, and then exhale, twisting to the left.

- Continue alternating sides for several rounds, gently massaging the spine and promoting flexibility.

c. *Seated Forward Bend:*
   - Your feet should be flat on the ground as you sit in the chair.

- Inhale and lengthen your spine.

- As you exhale, tilt forward from your hips and extend your hands toward the floor or your feet.

- Inhale as you lengthen your spine again, and then exhale, folding forward a bit deeper.

- Hold the pose for a few breaths, feeling the gentle stretch along the spine and hamstrings.

d. *Seated Cat-Cow Stretch:*
   - Sit tall and place your feet firmly on the ground.

- Inhale and arch your back, lifting your chest and chin (Cow Pose).

- Exhale, curve your back and tuck your chin into your chest to do the cat pose.

- Continue flowing between Cow and Cat Poses, focusing on the movement of your spine and breathing deeply.

4. **Breathing and Mindfulness:**
   Incorporate deep and mindful breathing techniques into your chair yoga practice. Focus on your breath during each pose, inhaling deeply and exhaling fully, to enhance relaxation and reduce pain-related tension.

5. **Listening to Your Body:**
   Always listen to your body and modify the poses as needed to suit your comfort level and pain tolerance. It's essential to avoid any movements

that may aggravate your pain.

6. **Consultation with Healthcare Professionals**:
Before starting a chair yoga practice for managing chronic pain, it is crucial to consult with healthcare professionals, such as a physician or physical therapist, to receive personalized guidance and ensure that the practice is suitable for your specific condition.

Heart Health and Circulation: Nurturing Cardiovascular Wellness from a Seated Position

Maintaining a healthy heart and circulation is essential for overall well-being and longevity. For individuals who may have limited mobility or find it challenging to engage in rigorous exercises, chair yoga offers a gentle yet effective way to support heart health and improve circulation. Chair yoga adapts traditional yoga poses for a seated or supported practice, making it accessible for individuals of all fitness levels. In this section, we will explore how chair yoga can benefit heart health and circulation, providing gentle movements and mindful practices to enhance cardiovascular wellness.

1. **The Importance of Heart Health and Circulation:**
A healthy heart and efficient circulation are crucial for delivering oxygen and nutrients throughout the body. Cardiovascular health plays a significant role in preventing heart disease and other related conditions.

2. **Understanding Chair Yoga for Heart Health:**
Chair yoga involves gentle stretches, breathing exercises, and relaxation techniques that can be performed while seated on a chair or using a chair for support. These practices help improve circulation, reduce stress, and support cardiovascular wellness.

3. **Chair Yoga Poses for Heart Health and Circulation:**
   a. *Seated Chest Opener:*
   - Sit tall on the chair with your feet flat on the floor.

- Interlace your fingers behind your back, opening your chest and shoulders.

- Lifting your chest upward while taking a deep breath.

- Exhale and release the stretch, relaxing your arms back to your sides.

- Repeat this movement a few times, focusing on opening the chest and enhancing breath capacity.

   b. *Seated Forward Bend*:
   - Put your feet flat on the floor and take a seat in the chair.

- Inhale and lengthen your spine.

- As you exhale, tilt forward from your hips and extend your hands toward the floor or your feet.

- Inhale as you lengthen your spine again, and then exhale, folding forward a bit deeper.

- Hold the pose for a few breaths, feeling the gentle stretch along the spine and hamstrings.

   c. *Seated Twist:*
   - Put your feet flat on the ground and take a comfortable seat.

- Inhale and lengthen your spine.

- Exhale and twist to the right, placing your left hand on your right knee and your right hand on the backrest of the chair.

- Inhale back to center, and then exhale, twisting to the left.

- Continue alternating sides for several rounds, gently massaging the spine and enhancing circulation.

4. **Breathing and Relaxation:**
   Incorporate deep breathing techniques, such as diaphragmatic breathing, into your chair yoga practice. Deep breaths help relax the body, reduce stress, and enhance circulation.

5. **Mindful Movement and Awareness:**
   Practice chair yoga with mindfulness and awareness of your body and breath. Focus on your heart center during heart-opening poses, fostering a sense of gratitude and compassion for your cardiovascular health.

6. **Consistency and Integration:**
   Consistent chair yoga practice is essential for experiencing the benefits for heart health and circulation. Integrate chair yoga into your daily routine, allowing it to become a mindful and rejuvenating practice.

7. **Consultation with Healthcare Professionals:**
   Before starting a chair yoga practice for heart health and circulation, it is crucial to consult with healthcare professionals, especially if you have any existing heart conditions or health concerns.

CHAPTER 5

Chair Yoga for Daily Living: Embracing Wellness and Mindfulness in Any Setting

Chair yoga offers a gentle and accessible way to incorporate yoga into our daily lives, regardless of age or physical abilities. The practice of chair yoga can be done in the comfort of a chair, making it convenient for various settings such as the office, home, or even while traveling. In this section, we will explore the benefits of chair yoga for daily living, simple chair yoga practices, and how it can be seamlessly integrated into your routine to promote well-being and mindfulness throughout the day.

1. **Benefits of Chair Yoga for Daily Living:**

   a. *Accessibility*: Chair yoga makes yoga accessible to individuals with mobility issues or those who find it challenging to practice traditional floor-based yoga.

b. *Improved Posture:* Regular practice of chair yoga can enhance posture by strengthening the core and supporting the spine.

c. *Stress Reduction:* Chair yoga incorporates breathing techniques and relaxation, promoting stress reduction and mental clarity.

d. *Enhanced Flexibility:* Gentle stretches and movements in chair yoga help improve flexibility, particularly in the neck, shoulders, and hips.

e. *Energizing:* Chair yoga can be invigorating, providing a burst of energy and revitalization, especially during long periods of sitting.

f. *Mindfulness:* The practice of chair yoga encourages mindfulness, helping individuals stay present and centered amidst their daily tasks.

2. **Simple Chair Yoga Practices:**
   a. *Seated Neck Stretches:*
   - Sit tall with your feet flat on the floor.

- As you breathe in, lengthen your spine.

- Exhale and tilt your head to the right, bringing your right ear towards your right shoulder.

- Inhale back to center, and then exhale, tilting your head to the left.

- Continue alternating sides for several rounds.

b. *Seated Shoulder Rolls:*
   - Take a comfortable seat with your feet flat on the ground.

- Breathe in as you raise your shoulders to your ears.

- Breathe out, then drop your shoulders.

- Continue this movement for several rounds, releasing tension in the neck and shoulders.

c. *Seated Spinal Twist*:
   - Sit tall and place your feet firmly on the ground.

- Inhale and lengthen your spine.

- Exhale and twist to the right, placing your left hand on your right knee and your right hand on the backrest of the chair.

- Inhale back to the center, and then exhale, twisting to the left.

- Continue alternating sides for several rounds, gently massaging the spine and improving flexibility.

d. *Seated Forward Bend*:
   - Put your feet flat on the ground and take a comfortable seat.

- Inhale and lengthen your spine.
   - Reach your hands toward your feet or the floor as you exhale and tilt forward from your hips.

- Inhale as you lengthen your spine again, and then exhale, folding forward a bit deeper.

- Hold the pose for a few breaths, feeling the gentle stretch along the spine and hamstrings.

3. **Integrating Chair Yoga into Daily Life:**
   a. *At the Office*: Take short breaks throughout the workday to practice

chair yoga stretches, releasing tension and revitalizing your body and mind.

b. *While Traveling*: Incorporate chair yoga practices during long flights or car rides to promote circulation and ease stiffness.

c. *At Home:* Make chair yoga a part of your morning or evening routine to start or end the day with mindfulness and relaxation.

d. *During Meetings or Waiting Times*: Use waiting periods or meetings to practice chair yoga breathing exercises, enhancing focus and calming the mind.

4. **Mindful Breathing**:

- Place your feet flat on the ground and take a comfortable seat in the chair.

- Lay your hands down on the floor with the palms facing up or down.

- Close your eyes or soften your gaze.

- Breathe deeply, using your nose to inhale and your mouth to exhale.

- Pay attention to the natural rhythm of your breath, feeling the rise and fall of your chest and abdomen.

- Stay in this mindful breathing practice for a few minutes, allowing yourself to be fully present in the moment.

Incorporating Chair Yoga into Your Daily Routine: Cultivating Wellness and Balance at Any Time

Chair yoga offers a versatile and accessible way to infuse wellness, relaxation, and mindfulness into your daily routine. Whether you're at the office, home, or on the go, chair yoga provides a convenient practice that can be tailored to your schedule and individual needs. In this section, we will explore practical tips and ideas for incorporating chair yoga into your daily routine, empowering you to embrace the transformative power of this gentle practice throughout the day.

1. **Create a Dedicated Space**:

Designate a quiet and comfortable space where you can practice chair yoga without distractions. Clear the area of clutter and create a calming atmosphere with soft lighting or natural light if possible.

2. **Set Aside Time:**

Identify specific times in your daily routine when you can integrate chair yoga seamlessly. Whether it's during your morning or afternoon break, while waiting for appointments, or before bedtime, find moments that work best for you.

3. **Start with Short Sessions:**

Begin with short chair yoga sessions, especially if you're new to the practice. A few minutes a day can make a significant difference in how you feel and can easily fit into your busy schedule.

4. **Incorporate Mindful Breathing**:

Use chair yoga as an opportunity to practice mindful breathing throughout the day. Whether you're at your desk, in a meeting, or commuting, take a few moments to focus on your breath and bring yourself into the present moment.

5. Utilize Breaks Wisely:

During work breaks, use chair yoga stretches and movements to release tension and revitalize your body and mind. Simple neck stretches, shoulder rolls, and seated twists can be done discreetly and effectively.

6. Engage in Desk Yoga:

While working at your desk, incorporate desk yoga postures to counter the effects of prolonged sitting. Perform seated forward bends, wrist stretches, and ankle circles to promote circulation and reduce stiffness.

7. Make Waiting Time Productive:

Use waiting times, such as in queues or before appointments, to practice chair yoga. Engage in mindful breathing, stretch your arms and legs, and gently twist your torso while waiting.

8. Wind Down with Evening Chair Yoga:

Before bedtime, unwind with gentle chair yoga poses that promote relaxation and prepare your body for rest. Gentle forward bends, seated twists, and mindful breathing can help you release the tensions of the day.

9. Customize Your Practice:

Tailor your chair yoga practice to address your specific needs and preferences. Whether you want to focus on relaxation, flexibility, or stress reduction, adapt the practice to suit your intentions.

10. Seek Guidance and Resources:

If you're new to chair yoga, consider seeking guidance from online resources, chair yoga classes, or instructional videos. Learning from experienced instructors can help you develop a safe and effective chair yoga practice.

Chair Yoga for Better Sleep: Cultivating Calmness and Relaxation Before Bedtime

Sleep is essential for overall well-being, and yet many people struggle with falling asleep or maintaining restful slumber. Incorporating chair yoga into your bedtime routine can be a gentle and effective way to promote relaxation, reduce stress, and prepare your body and mind for a restful night's sleep. In this section, we will explore chair yoga practices that can aid in better sleep, mindful breathing techniques, and tips for creating a bedtime ritual to enhance the quality of your sleep.

1. **The Importance of Sleep:**
   Sleep plays a vital role in the body's restoration and healing processes. Adequate and restful sleep contributes to improved cognitive function, emotional well-being, immune function, and overall vitality.

2. **How Chair Yoga Promotes Better Sleep:**
   Chair yoga before bedtime helps release tension from the body and calms the mind. The gentle stretches and mindful breathing activate the body's relaxation response, signaling to the nervous system that it's time to unwind.

3. **Chair Yoga Poses for Better Sleep:**
   a. *Seated Forward Bend:*
   - Put your feet flat on the ground and take a seat.

- Inhale and lengthen your spine.

- Reach your hands toward your feet or the floor as you exhale and tilt forward from your hips.

- Hold the pose for a few breaths, feeling the gentle stretch along the spine and hamstrings.

b. *Seated Twist:*
   - Put your feet flat on the ground and take a comfortable seat.

- Inhale and lengthen your spine.

- Exhale and twist to the right, placing your left hand on your right knee and your right hand on the backrest of the chair.

- Inhale back to center, and then exhale, twisting to the left.

- Continue alternating sides for several rounds, gently massaging the spine and promoting relaxation.

c. *Seated Neck Stretches:*
   - Sit tall and place your feet firmly on the ground.

- Inhale and lengthen your spine.

- Exhale and tilt your head to the right, bringing your right ear towards your right shoulder.

- Inhale back to center, and then exhale, tilting your head to the left.

- Continue alternating sides for several rounds, releasing tension in the neck and shoulders.

4. **Mindful Breathing for Better Sleep:**
   - Take a comfortable seat with your feet flat on the ground.

- Lay your hands down on the floor with the palms facing up or down.

- Shift your focus or avert your gaze.

- Take deep breaths, inhaling through your nose and exhaling through your mouth.

- Pay attention to the natural rhythm of your breath, feeling the rise and fall of your chest and abdomen.

- Focus on each breath, letting go of any thoughts or distractions that arise.

- Stay in this mindful breathing practice for a few minutes, allowing yourself to be fully present in the moment.

5. **Creating a Bedtime Ritual:**
   Establishing a calming bedtime ritual can signal to your body that it's time to unwind and prepare for sleep. Consider incorporating chair yoga, mindful breathing, or other relaxation practices into your bedtime routine. Other elements of a bedtime ritual might include:

- Dimming the lights to create a soothing environment.

- Reading a book or listening to calming music.

- Limiting screen time and exposure to electronic devices before bedtime.

- Sipping on a cup of caffeine-free herbal tea, such as chamomile or lavender, to promote relaxation.

Chair Yoga for Improved Posture: Strengthening the Core and Aligning the Spine

For general health and wellbeing, maintaining proper posture is crucial. However, the modern sedentary lifestyle and long hours of sitting can lead to poor posture and its associated discomforts. Chair yoga offers a gentle and effective way to improve posture by targeting the core muscles and aligning the spine. In this section, we will explore chair yoga poses and practices that can help strengthen the core, release tension in the back and shoulders, and cultivate better posture for a healthier and more aligned body.

1. **The Importance of Good Posture:**

Maintaining good posture not only enhances physical appearance but also plays a crucial role in preventing musculoskeletal issues and promoting optimal organ function. Proper posture helps distribute the body's weight evenly, reducing the strain on muscles and ligaments.

2. **How Chair Yoga Improves Posture:**

Chair yoga engages the core muscles, which are essential for supporting the spine and maintaining upright alignment. The practice of chair yoga also encourages awareness of body alignment and mindful movement, promoting better posture both during the practice and in everyday activities.

3. **Chair Yoga Poses for Improved Posture:**
   a. *Seated Mountain Pose:*
   - Place your feet flat on the floor while sitting tall on the chair.

- Maintain a straight spine, neck, and head position.

- Relax your shoulders and open your chest.

- Place your hands on your thighs or in a comfortable position on your lap.

- Breathe deeply and hold the pose for a few breaths, focusing on elongating your spine.

b. *Seated Cat-Cow Stretch*:
  - Sit up straight, feet flat on the ground.

- Inhale and arch your back, lifting your chest and chin (Cow Pose).

- As you exhale, curve your back and tuck your chin into your chest to do the cat pose.

- Continue flowing between Cow and Cat Poses, focusing on the movement of your spine.

c. *Seated Twist:*
  - Put your feet flat on the ground and take a comfortable seat.

- Inhale and lengthen your spine.

- Exhale and twist to the right, placing your left hand on your right knee and your right hand on the backrest of the chair.

- Inhale back to center, and then exhale, twisting to the left.

- Continue alternating sides for several rounds, gently massaging the spine and promoting better alignment.

d. *Seated Forward Bend*:
   - Put your feet flat on the ground and take a comfortable seat.

- Inhale and lengthen your spine.

- Reach your hands toward your feet or the floor as you exhale and tilt forward from your hips.

- Inhale as you lengthen your spine again, and then exhale, folding forward a bit deeper.

- Hold the pose for a few breaths, feeling the gentle stretch along the spine and hamstrings.

4. **Core-Strengthening Breathwork**:
   Deep breathing is not only essential for relaxation but also for engaging the core muscles. Practice diaphragmatic breathing, where you breathe deeply into your belly, engaging the core muscles as you inhale and relaxing them as you exhale.

5. **Mindful Posture Awareness:**
   Throughout the day, bring awareness to your posture during various activities, whether sitting, standing, or walking. Notice if your shoulders are hunched forward or if your spine is aligned, and make adjustments as needed.

Chair Yoga and Emotional Well-being: Nurturing Mind-Body Harmony for Inner Balance

Emotional well-being is a fundamental aspect of overall health, and it is intrinsically connected to our physical and mental state. Chair yoga offers a holistic approach to promoting emotional well-being by combining gentle physical movements, mindful breathing, and relaxation techniques. In this section, we will explore how chair yoga can positively impact emotional health, providing tools to manage stress, cultivate mindfulness, and foster a deeper connection between the body and mind.

1. **The Mind-Body Connection**:
   The mind-body connection emphasizes the interplay between our mental and physical states. Emotional well-being is influenced by the way we perceive and respond to life's experiences, and it can significantly impact our physical health and vice versa.

2. **How Chair Yoga Supports Emotional Well-being**:

a. *Stress Reduction:* Chair yoga incorporates relaxation techniques that activate the body's relaxation response, reducing stress hormones and promoting a sense of calmness.

b. *Mindfulness*: The mindful movements and breathwork in chair yoga cultivate present-moment awareness, helping individuals develop mindfulness and find grounding amidst daily challenges.

c. *Mood Enhancement*: Physical movements in chair yoga stimulate the release of endorphins, our body's natural mood enhancers, lifting spirits and promoting a positive outlook.

d. *Emotional Release*: Gentle movements and stretches in chair yoga can release physical tension, which may be associated with emotional holding, creating space for emotional release.

e. *Self-Compassion*: Chair yoga encourages self-compassion and non-judgmental awareness, supporting individuals in accepting and acknowledging their emotions without judgment.

3. **Chair Yoga Poses for Emotional Well-being**:
   a. *Seated Heart Opener:*
   - Place your feet firmly on the ground and sit tall in the chair.

- Place your hands on your lower back, fingers pointing down.

- Inhale and lift your heart towards the ceiling, gently arching your upper back.

- Exhale and release the stretch, coming back to a neutral position.

- Repeat the movement a few times, focusing on opening the chest and heart space.

b. *Seated Forward Bend:*
   - Place your feet flat on the floor and occupy the chair.

- Inhale and lengthen your spine.

- Reach your hands toward your feet or the floor as you exhale and tilt forward from your hips.

- Inhale as you lengthen your spine again, and then exhale, folding forward a bit deeper.

- Hold the pose for a few breaths, letting go of any tension and surrendering to the present moment.

c. *Seated Twist*:
   - Put your feet flat on the ground and take a comfortable seat.

- Inhale and lengthen your spine.

- Exhale and twist to the right, placing your left hand on your right knee and your right hand on the backrest of the chair.

- Inhale back to center, and then exhale, twisting to the left.

- Continue alternating sides for several rounds, breathing deeply and feeling the release of tension.

4. **Mindful Breathing and Meditation:**
Practice mindful breathing techniques during chair yoga, such as diaphragmatic breathing or 4-7-8 breathing, to promote relaxation and mindfulness. Incorporate short meditation sessions, focusing on the breath or cultivating positive emotions, to deepen the connection with your emotional well-being.

5. **Embrace Emotional Expression**:
Chair yoga provides a safe space to embrace and express emotions. Allow yourself to experience any emotions that arise during the practice without judgment or suppression.

CONCLUSION

In a world filled with constant demands and fast-paced living, it's easy to feel drained and disconnected from our own vitality. But what if there was a path that could lead us back to a life of energy, purpose, and joy? Welcome to where we invited you to embark on a transformative journey that nurtures your mind, body, and spirit through the gentle power of chair yoga.

Thank you from the depths of our hearts for embarking on this journey with "Chair Yoga for Seniors." Your dedication to exploring this gentle and transformative practice fills us with gratitude and joy.

We sincerely hope that you have found inspiration, empowerment, and renewed vitality within these pages. Your willingness to embrace the chair and embark on a path of well-being and self-discovery is truly admirable.

We humbly ask that you share your sincere feedback and leave a review for we will love to hear from you.

May each gentle movement and mindful breath you take on this chair yoga journey bring you closer to a life of grace, resilience, and ageless vitality. Remember that age should never limit your potential to lead a vibrant and fulfilling life.

As you continue to embrace the beauty of life with this practice, we wish you a heart overflowing with joy, a body filled with strength, and a spirit at peace. Thank you for being part of our community, and we hope this book has touched your life as profoundly as it has touched ours.